Getting Off the Couch

By

Robyn Job

Dedication

This book is dedicated to all the people who have transformed their lives under difficult circumstances, who have inspired the rest of us and showed us what can be done.

Contents

Introduction 1

CHAPTER 1: Who Are You? 4
   Activate Your Who 9

CHAPTER 2: Why Do You Want To Get Fit? 12
Short-Term Benefits 16
Long-Term Benefits 18
   Activate Your Why! 19

CHAPTER 3: Where Should You Train? 23
At Home 23
In a Gym 24
In a Fitness Class 25
In a Sport, Hobby or in General Activity 26
Mix it up 26
   Activate Your Where! 27

CHAPTER 4: What Do You Need To Do To Get Fit? 29
Cardiovascular Fitness 30
Resistance Training 30
Stretching and Balance 30
How Much is Enough? 31
Intensity Levels 33
Find your Base Movement 33
The Vigorous Zone 34
Putting It All Together 35
   Move 35
   Resistance: 35
   Intensify 36

What Keeps You Coming Back? 36
It's Individual 37
What is Your Motivation Level? **38**
Motivation Check-In 42

CHAPTER 5: How Do I Get Started And Stay The Distance? 44
Schedule it in! **44**
Activate Your Exercise Schedule! 45
Overcoming Guilt **47**
Finding Time **48**
Positive Affirmations **49**
Activate Your Positive Affirmations About Exercise: 50
Start Small **50**
Starting Staggered **52**
Overview **52**
1. Move: 53
2. Resist: 53
3. Intensify: 54
Walking Tips 55

CHAPTER 6: Epiphany Moments 56

CHAPTER 7: Workouts 58
Fitness Levels **59**
Beginners 59
Intermediate 60
Advanced 60
For Everyone 60
1. Home-Based No Equipment Circuit 1 ....**62**
2. Home-Based No Equipment Circuit 2 ....**65**
3. Home-Based Workout with Resistance Band Circuit 1 ....**68**
4. Home Based Workout with Resistance Band Circuit 2 ....**71**
Stretching **73**

CHAPTER 8: Training Schedules 76
1. Move (walk, cycle or swim) **78**
2. Resist: **84**
3. Intensify: **90**

CHAPTER 9: Re-Write Your Story..99
   Re-Activate Your Who 100

APPENDIX...102
 Heart Rate Zones...**102**
   Maximum Heart Rate ("MHR"):................................ 103
   Resting Heart Rate ("RHR") 103

About the Author...105

References...106

Introduction

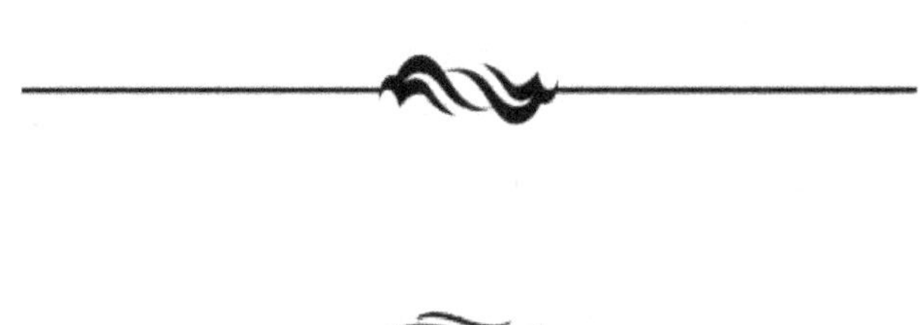

D o you want to get off the couch and cultivate an active lifestyle? Maybe you're busy and not spending much time on the couch at all; you're working, looking after the kids, multi-tasking and never getting time to sit down, let alone schedule a workout. If you are in one of these situations or anywhere in between, this book is designed to help you start— start where you're at and achieve the level of fitness that you can fit into your life right now.

There are already so many 'how to' books, apps, magazines, etc. on how and why to exercise. In this workbook, I'm going to share my journey and my own epiphany moments with the hope that it will inspire you to start your own journey into exercise. Making changes in our lives for the better is different for everyone, with some shared experiences.

The great thing is that the benefits of being fit are accessible to every person, regardless of background, personality or natural persuasion. My goal is to encourage you and help you see that consistent exercise can help you live better and live longer. By the way, if you believe you are really allergic to the word 'exercise', please feel free to substitute it throughout with 'activity'. ☺

This has been written in a 'workbook' style, so it is interactive, in order for you to understand some of your core beliefs and attitudes toward exercise. It's short because it's about action, not contemplation. Too much information and choices become paralysing, which just makes it harder to begin. And I assume you're reading this because you want to begin. So, let's start!

From herein, you'll find information and activities aimed at _you_ finding _your_ way to create an active life—one that will work for you in the long term. We'll look at:

1. Who you are when it comes to exercise

2. Why you want to be fit

3. Where you should get fit

4. What you need to do to get fit

5. How to get started and stay motivated

6. Epiphany moments

7. Workouts

8. Training schedules

CHAPTER 1

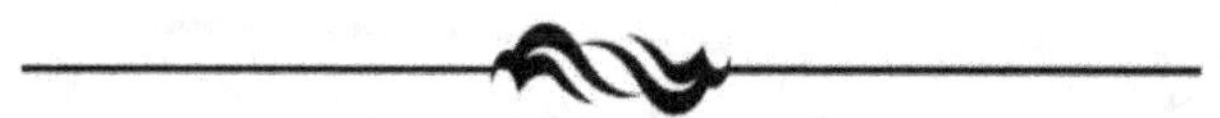

Who Are You?

What's your story? Your exercise background (or lack of it) affects the attitudes you have now. There may be things that happened in your past and upbringing that affect your feelings toward exercise—for good or for bad. Maybe you can identify some things as I share some of my own exercise journey.

In my family, running and being fit were highly valued. This is challenging if you're not naturally outdoorsy or sporty, like myself. My father was the instigator of this, being quite a serious long-distance runner in his teens and early 20s, and remaining active all his life. He often talked about running and being fit as something that was important; in doing so, he set the bar high! This put into motion a mindset that we all ought to be fit and exercising. My sister is also a natural runner like my father. As teenagers, when we went jogging together around our farm, she would be waiting for me at the top of the hill as I staggered up to catch my breath. My brothers were active with one inclined as a long-distance runner and one great at sprinting (eventually becoming a PE teacher and mamil [middle-aged male in lycra]). Even my mother at the age of 50 took up running half-marathons once a year for ten years and then 10km runs for eight years in a row.

At the annual high school cross country, most people walked, but I felt compelled to run (because no one walks in our family!). I would make a poor attempt at training for the event, knowing it would be the topic of conversation at the dinner table on the evening of the event. I usually came last in the sprinting on sports carnival day, felt intimidated in team sports and found volleyball terrifying. I did play soccer in my teens, which I loved. I often found myself in a game feeling like my lungs were on fire; it would have been more fun had I done some training in between games.

I put up a good front, but on the inside, I felt like the black sheep of the exercising family.

When I then moved away to the city at 19 years of age... all the external reasons ('pressure') to exercise were gone! Occasionally, I would get questions from my family like, "What sport are you playing?" It was still subtle pressure but far enough away for me to sweep it under the carpet. But, in the back of my mind, I always knew that exercise was important, and I was always going to start someday, I just hadn't gotten around to it yet.

And somehow, someday, I did start... 15 years later. But, before this, I had my bouts of trying and failing, such as starting a jogging regime or joining a gym and getting a program, signing up for the gym with a friend and getting a program, doing an aerobics class and getting injured; all of which amounted to a couple of weeks at most. It just wouldn't stick. I didn't know why. I would berate myself for not having enough willpower while I found valid excuses not to continue.

In my early 30s, I had begun contemplating getting fit (again). My flatmate was going overseas for three weeks. For me, this was the magical time frame I believed I would need to exercise in order to 'see a difference'. I purchased a videotape of a workout I could do at home. While she was away, I knew the TV would be mine—I would be able to come home from work and put on that video without anyone watching me. I would be unimpeded to get on and do it. So, I did. I stuck to the plan. That was the start. I also started walking after work in the summer, along the beautiful Coogee-Clovelly coastline. It wasn't terribly consistent or scheduled in, but I was getting active.

When a friend gave me a free ticket to the 'Fitness Expo' in Sydney, I was curious. I went along, getting inspired by the various exhibitions and talks. But then I stumbled upon the Body for Life exhibition. I got into a conversation with a remarkably fit 'Body for Lifer'. I was so inspired by the idea of three months of transformation with a food and exercise program. I was given a videotape telling the stories of the finalists from the first Body for Life competition. Not being from the fitness industry, I had never seen anything like it. I thought the transformations were quite extraordinary. I was brimming with motivation. After some reflection and mulling over for the next few days, somewhere deep inside, I made a decision to 'go for it! '. I purchased the book and read it from cover to cover so I knew what was in store. I told friends and family that I was going to do it... I got organised so that I had all the right food at hand and had access to a local gym. In order not to 'fail' on the first week, I set up a 'practice week' so that I knew when/what the challenging things would be. If I stuffed up in the practice week, it wasn't really failing. I wanted to start strong. It was a great strategy that worked well for me psychologically.

One of the things I needed to do to get organised was to inform my two flatmates at the time that I wouldn't be collaborating with them on the weekly food shopping/cooking. For the next three months, I would be eating Body for Life-style. They were very quick to say that they would like to do it with me. That was one problem solved and certainly made it a lot easier with the household eating the same way and with less tempting food in the house. A group of friends (three guys) in a house nearby also decided to do the Body for Life challenge. It was, again, helpful to have the support of friends and people around me who were interested in what I was doing and even doing it too.

Surprisingly, I was very motivated and stuck to the program 90-95%. I remember feeling quite hungry before meals for the first three weeks, but after that, my mind and body adjusted. I toned up and went down two dress sizes. People who hadn't seen me in the three-month period were surprised at the change. It was a new direction in life for me. I had discovered fitness and wanted to tell everyone about its benefits. I had more energy and noticed that even if I didn't sleep well, I could cope better the next day. It helped me to quite dramatically reduce and get rid of tension headaches— something I hadn't anticipated. My body image and confidence improved. I wasn't perfect but I knew that I was doing the best I could, and just wasn't so self-conscious anymore. This was very freeing. I felt like an overcomer, which helped in other areas of my life.

So, whether it's weightlifting and cardio at the gym, or walking and Pilates from home, I have never looked back from that point on. I am committed to being a long-term exerciser. I had experienced too many benefits to turn back.

Some people have quite extraordinary transformations; they've lost 20kg or gone from crutches to running. In comparison, my story is quite ordinary, however, I got 'off the couch' (got started) and am healthier for it. I know from first-hand experience that it can be hard to start, to break bad habits and carve out good ones. So, any time we make long-term changes for the better, it's a victory!

What is your experience? Have you started and stopped exercise programs and never managed to make them last long-term? Have you had bad experiences? Or maybe you have been super fit in the past and now find yourself unfit and feeling it. Whatever your situation is, let's find the spark to get you going in the right direction.

Activate Your Who

Who are you when it comes to exercise? If it was a relationship, how would you describe it? Circle one word below that fits you best right now:

Unacquainted	Distant acquaintance	Casual friendship
Friend	Close friend	Long-term relationship
	It's complicated!	

Below (or in a notebook), take a few minutes to think about your relationship with exercise, activity or sport. Have there been moments of inspiration and success; moments of giving up and getting despondent? How did you feel growing up about exercise? How do you feel now?

____

____

____

CHAPTER 2

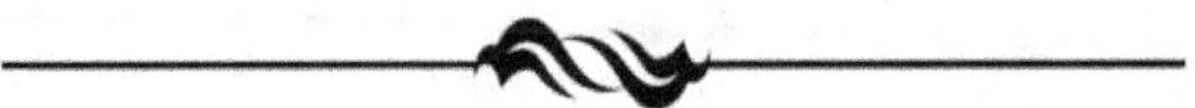

Why Do You Want To Get Fit?

Why Should You Get More Active?

The couch is comfortable! Unless you have a good reason to get out of your current comfort zone, why would you? If your life is more in the 'busy zone', you may think, "How can I add more to my schedule?" Exercise has loads of benefits, but not exercising ('not being active') has many negative consequences to our physical, mental and emotional wellbeing. Perhaps you are experiencing some of them right now.

Conduct an interview with yourself using the table below (or in a workbook). Brainstorm all your reasons for and against exercise. This may sound counterproductive, but it's a good exercise to see where the payoffs of exercise may be for you.

Box 1 - Benefits of Staying the Same

(Ask yourself: "What is something *good* about not choosing to get active?")

This might include things you currently love doing and would need to sacrifice, such as reducing reading time or missing a favourite TV show to attend a fitness class. Perhaps your only time to exercise is in the morning and you love sleeping in. The benefits of not exercising are that you get to keep/do all these things.

Box 2 - Concerns About Staying the Same

(Ask yourself: "What is something *bad* that could happen if I do stay the same?")

For example, some people say they hide in family photos because they don't like the way they look. They live with the anxiety of this. Getting active may increase body confidence and self-esteem and lessen your anxiety over these things. Doing nothing will mean this concern remains in your life.

Box 3 – Concerns About the Change

(Ask yourself: "What is something *bad* that could come from making the change?")

For example, you may live near a busy road, so walking may mean you are breathing in fumes or contending with noisy traffic. Perhaps you fear snakes, spiders and leeches and are afraid to go bushwalking!

Box 4 – Reasons to Change

(Ask yourself: "What is something *good* that could come from taking action to get active?")

There are many benefits of exercise. These are the results you are expecting from exercise. It might be better health, improved bone density, being able to play with grandkids or go on a three-day hike.

Brainstorm away with the table below!

1. Benefits of staying the same	2. Concerns about staying the same
3. Concerns about change	**4. Reasons to change**

Now, let's focus on the benefits:

Short-Term Benefits

One of the problematic mindsets I had to getting started with exercise was that I would only see results "way in the future". I was told it would be "three weeks" before I'd see any difference and that would be small. As a non-exerciser at the time, this seemed like a long time I had to get hot and sweaty to see minor results. However, I was wrong, there are some AMAZING immediate benefits to exercise. I would even call it *instant*, and who doesn't love 'instant gratification'! Check out this list: [1]

- **<u>Endorphins</u>**. During and after exercise, endorphins are released that make you feel good!   Beware, you may even feel as if you can 'take on the world' after an exercise session!

- **<u>Clears the mind</u>**. After a workout, many problems of the day do not seem so 'unsolvable' anymore. It kind of 'clears the cobwebs' of the mind. This is especially so with cardio (huff and puff) exercise. Our ability to think is enhanced because the chemistry of the brain is altered; hormones and enzymes are recruited to keep the body in balance.

---

[1] https://www.sciencedirect.com/science/article/pii/S0378512217308563

- **<u>*Creates focus*</u>.** Whether you're focusing on your form or counting your reps, exercise can become a type of mindfulness where you change your attention from problems and concerns to be "in the present moment". Needless to say, this is great for mental health!

- **<u>*Stress melts away*</u>.** In our busy lifestyles, tension can often build up as our day goes on. Exercise helps to relax tense muscles. This can have many benefits, such as minimizing headaches, preventing further neck and shoulder issues and generally being a better person to live with.

- **<u>YOU-*time*</u>.** Make exercise your time to process life and take some time out for yourself. It's your daily dose of 'you-time'.

Long-Term Benefits

While you're enjoying the instant benefits of exercise, you can start looking forward to the longer-term benefits:

- **<u>Improved appearance</u>** by toning and shaping the body.

- **<u>Improved circulation and complexion</u>**. Who needs expensive skin care creams? Exercise nourishes the skin over your entire body by increasing the circulation of fresh blood, oxygen, and nutrients. Additionally, it helps draw toxins out of the body and improve the condition of the outer layer of your skin.

- **<u>Weight loss</u>**. Exercise burns fat and increases metabolism, which helps with weight management.

- **<u>Look younger</u>**. Look and feel younger as exercise helps reverse and slow down the aging process.

- **<u>Boosts confidence and self-esteem</u>**. There is something that rises up within you when you have become a long-term, committed exerciser; a sense of personal power of your endurance, strength and flexibility. Additionally, the discipline you are creating through this area of your life will spill over into other areas.

- **<u>Build immunity</u>**. It increases the immune system because it increases your white blood cell count.

- **<u>Reduce heart disease</u>.** Exercise increases the good cholesterol and decreases the bad, making it a great way of managing heart disease.

- **<u>Ward off dementia</u>.** Cardio (aerobic) style exercise can be protective against developing dementia.[2]

- **<u>Stay independent</u>.** Exercise increases your flexibility and, therefore, range of motion. This is great as it can help you to hang onto your independence as you age. We lose muscle mass as we age but activity can help bring back flexibility, balance and strength of muscles.

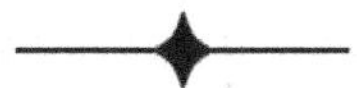

Activate Your Why!

Now it's time to activate *your* reasons for wanting to get active. This is one of the most important things you can do to get started and become a consistent exerciser. If it's not a strong enough reason, it's more difficult to stay motivated during hard times. A strong reason is often connected to *emotions*. Below is a list of many of the benefits of exercise, both long and short-term categorised under types of exercise. As you read this list, take note of what 'sparks' inspiration for you:

---

[2] https://www.sciencedirect.com/science/article/pii/S0025619611652191

Benefits of Resistance Training
<ul><li>Assists weight loss (by increasing muscle mass and raising metabolic rate)</li><li>Prevention from injury</li><li>Rehabilitation from injury</li><li>Better posture and more toned appearance</li><li>Increase in confidence and self-esteem</li><li>Increases strength, speed, power, muscular endurance and physical performance (i.e. generally and in sports activities)</li><li>Increases bone density</li><li>Helps reverse the aging process by reversing muscle loss</li></ul>
Benefits of Cardio Exercise
<ul><li>Fit to do the things you want to (e.g., a sport, bushwalking)</li><li>Increases energy to get through the day</li><li>Improves mood and wards off depression</li><li>Reduces stress and tension</li><li>Reduces risk of stroke and heart disease</li><li>Assists in weight loss</li></ul>
Benefits of Stretching and Balance
<ul><li>Prevention of falls allows you to stay independent longer</li></ul>
<ul><li>Increases range of motion of joints, helping to prevent injuries and aid rehabilitation.</li></ul>
<ul><li>Improves wellness, mindfulness and focus.</li></ul>

As you can see, there are many fabulous reasons to exercise from external (how you look), internal (confidence), physical (energy), mental (wellbeing) or preventative (health and longevity). These ideas are just to get your mind and emotions stimulated. There are many other valid reasons to get active that may be completely unique to you. Using the list above and/or adding your own reasons, write down the main paybacks you want from exercise below (or in a workbook).

Choose one *overriding* reason from the list above; the one that brings up the *most* emotion for you:

My overriding and compelling reason to become more active is:

____

____

____

If you're not sure, don't despair! Sometimes we only know the benefits by starting. I got way more benefits than I anticipated before I began. One lady, who did no other exercise but attend my Pilates class once a week, was able to stop taking painkillers for her back pain. I'm sure she did not expect such amazing results from one class per week. If you're still not convinced, I encourage you to start and take note of how you feel after one workout session, after three weeks and then after three months!

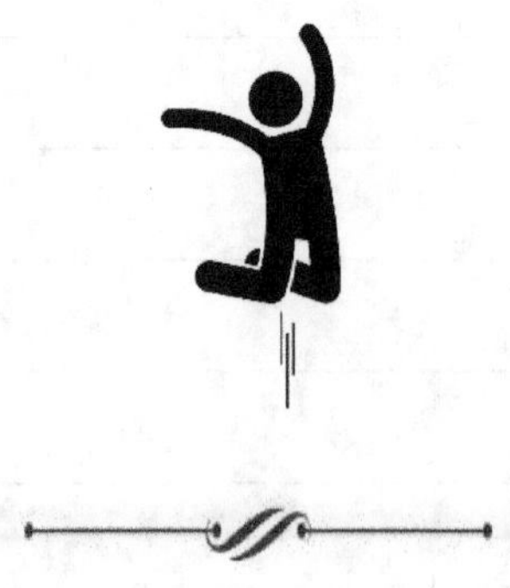

CHAPTER 3

Where Should You Train?

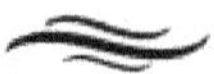

There's no right or wrong 'venue' to train in, you just find the place that works best for you.

At Home

If you're definitely not a "gym person", that's ok! You can start training simply and cheaply from home. All you need is a good pair of walking/jogging shoes that will support your feet and cushion your joints. When you've got the walking down pat, you can add some home-based resistance exercises. There are some walking tips and sample exercises in Chapter 7 of this book that can get you started.

Advantages of exercising at home are that it's free (unless you purchase expensive equipment from an infomercial!). You can do quite a lot with no equipment or with some very inexpensive gear. However, there can be distractions, a lack of space, and it can be demotivating working out alone. You will only know if it's right for you once you give it a try.

In a Gym

A gym is a great place to exercise to either enhance your home-based workouts or instead of it. It can be intimidating going to a gym for the first time, but there is usually someone you can book a time with to help you.

I understand that, for some, the gym is not a 'natural' environment. It's true that, back in the day, those living off the land, without modern conveniences, did not *need* a gym. In cultures where there is a higher-than-average percentage of people reaching 100 (in good health), they live a naturally active lifestyle. This includes simple everyday activities like walking, gardening, washing and chopping firewood. What we've done now, with modern living (cars, washing machines, mix masters, vacuum cleaners, chain saws) is eliminate a lot of the activity that would naturally keep us moving more. Now, while you put your washing on to agitate the clothes, you can sit down with a cup of tea and a biscuit. My grandmother had a hand wringer for her clothes. There's your bicep day right there! Going to the gym is a way of adding that activity back in. Really, I see the gym like a playground full of swings and roundabouts, a jumping castle that I can't wait to dive into and start working up a sweat. I didn't always feel that way! So, while you don't need to go to a gym, please consider giving it a try before you make your final decision to work out what's best for you.

In a Fitness Class

When you attend a gym, you are most likely surrounded by people but possibly working out on your own, doing your own program. This suits some people just fine (usually the introverts). In fitness classes, you are working with a group and an instructor. Many people find this more motivating than attending the gym on their own (unless they can find a reliable 'workout buddy').

Fitness classes offer great connection with others, accountability and motivation. There's such a variety that you can usually find one that is your 'style'. They range from calming yoga and Pilates to energetic spin bike and Zumba classes. The question is, what is available in your area and at a time that suits you? If you think this style of exercise is your thing, take a step into action by finding out what's available near you.

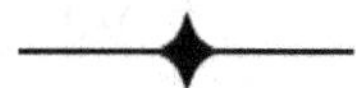

In a Sport, Hobby or in General Activity

Repetitive exercise is not for everyone. There are other ways to get active, such as playing a sport, joining a bushwalking group, dancing, golfing, cycling or riding to work, taking the stairs, or taking up rollerblading. These are great ways to get fit, but keep in mind the recommendations outlined in the next chapter so that you get your activity levels up to the point of getting all the benefits.

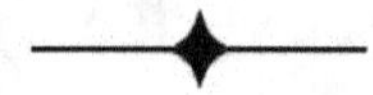

Mix it up

Get creative! Perhaps you can fit in a round of golf to get your walking in one day a week; a spin class for your vigorous exercise, and some home-based workouts and one gym session. Variety will prevent boredom and feeling like you're stuck in a routine.

Activate Your Where!

Take some time to fill out the questions below (or in a notebook).

Activities I have liked/loved previously are:

(E.g., I really enjoyed attending the fitness class.)

Activities I have loathed previously are:

(E.g., I didn't like the smell of the gym but maybe I can get over that.)

I would like to begin exercising at/by:

(E.g., I would like to check out the local fitness class and bushwalking group.)

____

____

Great, that's a good start! You may change your mind later, but you need a direction to begin with. If you're still not sure, you can check out the walking plan and sample workouts in Chapter 7.

CHAPTER 4

What Do You Need To Do To Get Fit?

To reap the benefits of exercise mentioned above, there are some recommendations to aim for. These are outlined below. However, it's ok to start where you can and build up from there. It's important to avoid an 'all or nothing' mindset because when it comes to exercise: *Something is better than nothing* and *perfectionism breeds inactivity.*

If you are new to the world of exercise, there are <u>three</u> main components to fitness. It's great if you can combine all three in your workouts or over a weekly period. These are:

Cardiovascular Fitness – This is fitness for the heart and lungs. It is the kind of exercise that will get you 'huffing and puffing' and raise your heart rate. This includes walking, swimming, cycling, running, various gym cardio equipment such as treadmills, bikes, cross trainers, steppers and playing heart-raising sports such as tennis, soccer and touch footy.

Resistance Training – This is fitness for the muscles. It can include lifting weights such as dumbbells and using weight machines, body weight exercises, Pilates, yoga, elastic band, fit ball exercises and much more... any type of exercise where you are putting resistance on the muscles. Resistance causes the muscles to grow in size but the size of this growth will vary depending on the type of resistance training, how heavy you lift and other factors.

Stretching and Balance – Stretching at the end of a workout is a great way to treat yourself as it feels very restorative. It will increase the range of motion in your joints. The ability to balance diminishes as we get older. Whatever age you are, why not start practicing now by including it in your resistance training session?

You can also fit balance into your daily activities, such as standing on one leg for 30 seconds when you are in a queue or brushing your teeth. Find creative ways to fit balance into your day.

How Much is Enough?

Current guidelines for adults (18 to 64 years of age) are:[3]

Cardio Exercise:

We can either do:

> ➢ 2.5 to 5 hours of moderate activity

> OR

> ➢ 1.25 to 2.5 hours of vigorous activity

As you can see, you can do less activity if it is more intense. Another option is to combine moderate and vigorous exercises. For best results, try to exercise each day, or without too many days' gap in between.

Resistance Exercise:

> ➢ Current guidelines recommend a minimum of two resistance sessions per week for all major muscle groups.

---

[3] https://www.health.gov.au/health-topics/physical-activity-and-exercise/physical-activity-and-exercise-guidelines-for-all-australians/for-adults-18-to-64-years:

Upper Body	Lower Body	Core
Chest, back, shoulders and arms (biceps and triceps)	Quadriceps (front of thighs) Hamstrings (back of thighs) Can also include glutes and calves	Abdominals

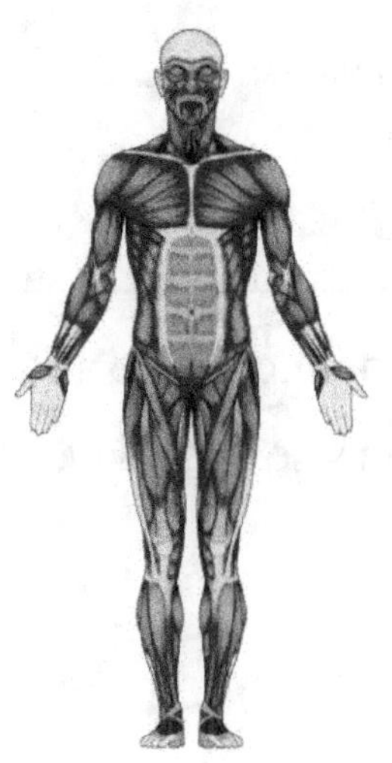 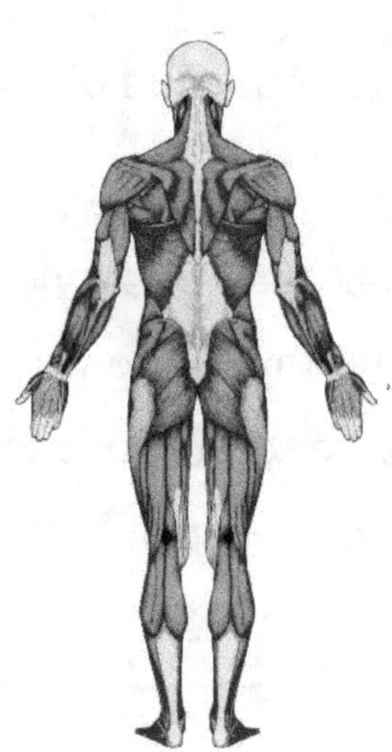

Intensity Levels

Below is an indication of how to tell what level of intensity you are performing in your workout:

❖ *Low* = heart rate & breathing not increased. *Able to hold a conversation and sing a song.*

❖ *Moderate* = mildly increased heart rate and breathing. *Able to talk but not sing.*

❖ *High* = sweating and increased heart rate and breathing. *Not able to talk except for a word or two.*

If you'd like to get more technical about intensity levels, see the heart rate section in the appendix.

Find your Base Movement

When you are starting to work up to your 2.5 hours of moderate-intensity exercise, it's helpful to identify your 'base' movement. Something accessible and without too many barriers. For most people, this will be walking and perhaps cycling or swimming. Walking is a great place to start because it can stop the decline of lower limb bone density.[1&2] Cycling and swimming do not have as many benefits for bone density but may be easier on the joints. You could always try a mixture of two or three. Resistance training will also be beneficial for bone density, so you will not be missing out altogether if you choose cycling or swimming.

The Vigorous Zone

Vigorous exercise is great for your health as it is considered more heart-protective than moderate exercise.[4]

There is more than one way to exercise to get your heart rate up into the vigorous zone. You may have heard of terms like 'fast exercise' and 'High-Intensity Interval Training' (HIIT). This means doing short bursts of intense exercise that raise your heart rate substantially, so much so that you couldn't keep it up for more than 20-60 seconds. In comparison, there is 'steady-state' cardio, which is the type of movement you can sustain for longer periods, e.g., up to 45 mins. There are benefits of HIIT and steady-state exercise, so it's good to include both in your weekly workout schedule.

[4] https://pubmed.ncbi.nlm.nih.gov/16377300/ Swain DP, Franklin BA. Comparison of cardioprotective benefits of vigorous versus moderate intensity aerobic exercise. Am J Cardiol. 2006 Jan 1;97(1):141-7. doi: 10.1016/j.amjcard.2005.07.130. Epub 2005 Nov 16. PMID: 16377300.

Putting It All Together

How do you put this into action?

Move: If you walk, cycle or swim for 30 minutes a day, five times a week, this will add up to 2.5 hours of moderate exercise. You can check if you are in the moderate zone using the scale above, or by a simple heart rate calculation (see the appendix).

ADD: Stretching at the end of your workout.

Resistance: Two 'resistance' sessions of all major muscle groups could be done as follows:

- Two at-home or gym workouts on two days per week (separated by 48 hours), OR,

- Attending two resistance-based classes a week, OR,

- Four x 30 minutes sessions breaking down the major muscle groups, e.g., two upper body days, two lower body days.

ADD: Balance (and stretching) into or at the end of resistance training.

Intensify: Your base movement can be used to introduce your higher-intensity exercise when you get to that point. For example, adding some hills into your walk or increasing it to a jog or intermittent jog/walk. Similarly, with cycling or swimming, you can add some faster-paced bursts. If/when you reach the vigorous intensity zone, you can decrease the amount of 'minutes' you are doing, making your workout sessions more time-efficient.

Maybe you have some fitness goals or play a sport that will require you to train more in the vigorous zone.

What Keeps You Coming Back?

The main aim with your exercise is to choose something that you will look forward to rather than find excuses not to do. You need the type of activity that will keep you coming back for more. It might take a bit of 'trial and error' to start with. It doesn't mean that there will be some days that you don't feel like going, but you can still convince yourself to do it.

I attended a very intense, one-hour, early morning circuit class at a gym I belonged to for a while. Eventually, I couldn't bring myself to go. Although I was quite fit at the time, it wasn't sustainable for me. I prefer moderate-intensity with short bursts of vigorous exercise. According to the latest science, that's ok; it doesn't have to be constant, high-intensity exercise to get the benefits. Eventually, I stopped going to the class, but there were regulars there that kept going week in, week out. It was fine for them, but I had to find something else. It's important to choose an activity that will keep _you_ coming back.

It's Individual

The type and intensity of exercise can be quite an individual thing. You may want to start with low-intensity and move to a higher intensity level when you have been exercising for a while. There are people out there that love intense exercise! Others would be turned off for life by super intense, heart-raising exercise. Before my Body for Life challenge, I was fairly unacquainted with getting hot and sweaty. I avoided it at all costs. I am now quite ok with that and actually miss it if I've gone for a few days without a 'cardio fix'. So, like wine, olives and yoghurt, it's an acquired taste that you can learn to love, or at least get used to it as a part of your life. You don't brush your teeth because you love it, but you know it has benefits if you do it and drawbacks if you don't. Exercise can be like that.

While you can start with low-intensity, it's beneficial to get into the moderate zone, and some vigorous if and when you can. But if that isn't 'you' to start with, don't let that stop you. Start with something and build up to some short spurts of vigorous exercise.

The simplest way to get your cardio workout in is to put on a pair of joggers and head out the door!

It's ok to try out a few things to find what works for you. While it's great to aim for a time-efficient weights workout, the best exercise is one that keeps you coming back. Consistency is the key. Consistency gets you results.

What is Your Motivation Level?

Are you truly ready to begin?

See if you can identify yourself in one of these stages:

Stage	What you can do if you're in this stage:
Pre-contemplation – You are not considering making any change. Perhaps a family member or GP has suggested you make changes but you	Keep reading and fact-finding about the benefits of exercise because the drawbacks do outweigh the benefits. Read inspirational

see more of the drawbacks than the benefits. E.g., A family member is concerned about your health. You are only reading this book because they gave it to you and you promised them you would read it. 😊	stories and scientific articles. Consider your health. As a non-exerciser, I think we probably go in and out of this phase. Often not thinking about exercise at all, and then we overhear something or are confronted with a health issue, and the topic of exercise arises again.
Contemplation – you know there is need for change and are thinking about things. The drawback and benefits are about equal to you. E.g., Thinking you don't have time to exercise but it would be good to lose a bit of weight. You're telling yourself you need to get fit but not taking any action toward it.	It's awesome you're considering getting active and looking into the benefits. Keep researching the benefits, get inspired, journal your barriers, ask for help.
Decision – You are ready to do something within the next month or so. You are taking steps toward making that happen. At this point, you are convinced that the benefits outweigh the drawbacks. E.g., You've made enquiries about prices and classes at the local gym.	Great, you've decided to get fit! Plan for success. You're motivated and excited to get started; don't bite off more than you can chew to start with. The more organised you are, the more likely you are to succeed.

Action – You are taking action and changing your behaviour, getting rid of bad habits and replacing them with good ones. E.g., You've committed to walking with a friend for three mornings a week and are doing it.	You've started! Stay 'behaviour modification alert', i.e. how is it working in your schedule? What needs to be tweaked so that this is a long-term venture?
Maintenance – You have been living out your new healthy lifestyle for at least six months and intend to keep going. E.g., You've taken out a six-month gym membership and are telling everyone how much you love being fit and are noticing the difference in your life.	Wow, look at you now! Claim this new person as your new identity: "I am a committed long-term exerciser." "I love exercising."
Relapse – You have slipped back into old habits. You may or may not intend to return to the healthier habits. E.g., You had an injury or illness that stopped you exercising for a long period. You're now finding it difficult to find the motivation to start again.	It happens! That's why there's a section for it. Start doing something as soon as you can. You might need to start small again. Maybe you need a change and to try something new. If you went overseas on a holiday and got out of the rhythm of exercising, get back into it as soon as you can.

When I think about my own journey, I went in and out of pre-contemplation and contemplation for many years. If a family member asked me about sports or exercise, or I thought I was putting on weight, etc., I would go into contemplation and then slip back again into not thinking about exercise.

I was in the decision stage when I planned and bought the videotape for the three weeks my flatmate was away. Before the Body for Life challenge, I read the book, looked at the video and talked to my flatmates about food. This planning was setting me up for success. Even though you haven't started in the 'Decision' stage, don't underestimate the power of planning and setting yourself up to win.

Before the Body for Life challenge, in my first attempts at exercise (e.g., joining a gym for a few weeks), I did not stay long enough to get into the 'Maintenance' stage. This is important because if we stick at it long enough, we WANT to keep exercising.

The initial three-month program allowed me to stick at it long enough to experience the benefits and stay around long-term.

Although I have never had any long-term relapses, I have had times when I've found it difficult to get into the vigorous zone. This requires pushing yourself out of the comfort zone which is always one of the hardest things to do exercise-wise. Every now and then, I need to have a talk with myself and remind myself of the benefits! I heard a professional female bodybuilder use the phrase once: "Don't spend too long out of the saddle." In other words, if you take a week off, get back into your workout routine as soon as you can. The longer you leave it, the less motivated you will be. After times of injury and illness, you may not be able to get back to where you were, but if you do what you can, you can feel good about what you are doing.

Now, think about where you are at and answer the question below (or in a notebook):

Motivation Check-In

I can identify with _________________________________ stage above.

Based on this understanding, I am going to take action by:

____

____

____

I will do this by: ______ /_______ /_________.

CHAPTER 5

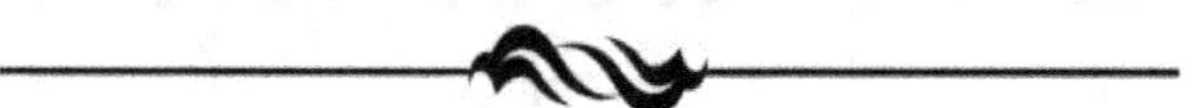

How Do I Get Started And Stay The Distance?

S et yourself up for success by implementing these strategies:

Schedule it in!

One tip to be successful with exercise is to schedule some time each week. Decide how much time you can 'afford'. Time is like money and needs to be budgeted wisely. Be realistic and allow buffer time before and after.

Scheduling in and planning workout times will help it to become a habit. Motivation is what gets us started, but habit keeps us going.

Choosing the right time to exercise can depend on:

- When you have free time (e.g., if you work, look after the kids, volunteer, etc.)

- When you have more energy (am or pm)

- When the gym/pool is open

- When classes are scheduled or when your workout buddy is free.

Exercising in the morning is great because it prioritises it and makes sure it gets done. However, exercising toward the end of the day is a great stress release. What are you best times?

Activate Your Exercise Schedule!

Circle your best time to exercise:

Morning   Mid-morning   Midday

Mid-afternoon   Evening

Perhaps each day is different. Try to identify where you can find time to schedule workouts in your week using the chart below:

Time	Mon	Tues	Wed	Thurs	Fri	Sat	Sun
5 am							
6 am							
7 am							
8 am							
9 am							
10 am							
11 am							
12 pm							
1 pm							
2 pm							
3 pm							
4 pm							
5 pm							
6 pm							
7 pm							
8 pm							
9 pm							
10 pm							

Don't be discouraged if you don't have a lot of time. A 20-30-minute resistance session is a great place to start! Ten minutes of activity three times a day can also be a great aim. For example, doing some squats while you wait for the kettle to boil, or during the ad breaks. You can schedule this in also, and tick it off when you've done it.

Overcoming Guilt

Are you busy looking after other people and have no time for yourself? Remember that energy begets energy. When you expend energy exercising, you create more energy to expend elsewhere. Taking a little time for exercise might give you extra energy and clarity of thinking to help you push through other tasks. In airplanes, they tell you in an emergency to put the oxygen mask on yourself first before your children. Your first thought might be, "That sounds selfish," but when you think about it, it's very logical. You can't help anyone else if you run out of oxygen. You can benefit those around you when you have more energy, think with more clarity, are less stressed, get sick less often and you feel better about yourself. The oxygen analogy is good to keep in mind.

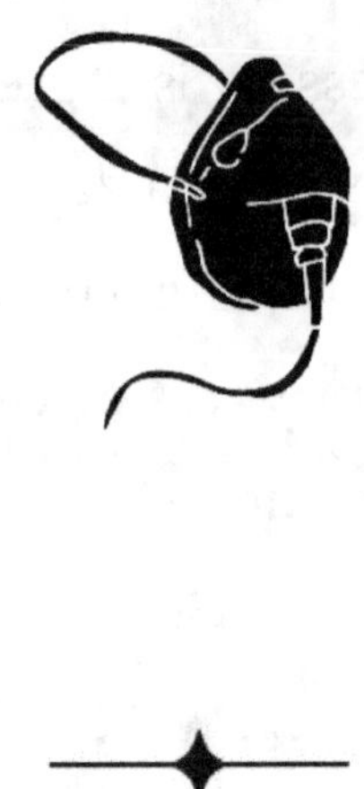

Finding Time

If you are working full-time, don't despair. I found that I did more exercise and was more consistent when I worked full-time. I think it comes down to, "If you want to get something done, give it to a busy person." Ironically, it is much harder for me to find time working part-time in a gym! I like to think of "tucking" exercise into the beginning or end of the day, i.e. before or after work. Some people try their lunch hour. The idea behind "tucking in" exercise is that you are not dedicating a 'whole morning' or 'whole afternoon' to it. The key is to find a slot of time that works for you and *protect* that time. Make it non-negotiable if someone wants to steal it from you!

If you can, aim for exercising most days of the week rather than a big chunk on the weekend. But as always, something is better than nothing.

Positive Affirmations

Thoughts are the seeds that shape our lives. How you think about exercise will, in the end, determine whether you will be motivated to do it, or not.

Become a thought detective and start replacing your negative thoughts about exercise with positive ones. Some examples are below, but it's good to come up with some that will work for you:

- Exercise gives me so much energy

- My mind feels so clear after I exercise

- I look forward to my workout

- I feel so great after my workout

- I know this is reversing the aging process

- I know this is preventing my headaches / insomnia / _ _ _ _ _ _ ?

- I'm going to exercise for the rest of my life because I love it

- I can't wait to get to the gym and release the tension of the day.

Activate Your Positive Affirmations About Exercise:

- ____

- ____

- ____

- ____

- ____

- ____

- ____

Start Small

If jumping into a one-hour-a-day workout regime makes you feel like you've joined the SAS, you're not crazy and you're not alone. Starting small and simple will create a habit that you can build on. James Clear in 'Atomic Habits'[5] recommends making it so simple, you can't say no. For example, starting with a five-minute walk, or one push-up, or just stretching. Inspire yourself to the next level, rather than reprimand yourself there.

The first time I attempted a one-hour spin class, I didn't know what hit me. I put on a brave face to keep up with everyone else in the class, but inwardly, I was dying. I was dripping with sweat, couldn't catch my breath and exhausted well before the end of the class. I was planning on not going back, but after a conversation with another participant, I realised I could drop in for the first 20-30 minutes. I started doing that regularly and, eventually, was able to do the whole class. I did feel like a member of the SAS by the end of the class, but I had to work up to that. Here is some ancient wisdom: "Do not despise small beginnings" (Zech 4v10). Check with the instructor first, if there are options or ways to 'ease into' the class.

---

[5] Clear, J. (2018). *Atomic habits: tiny changes, remarkable results : an easy & proven way to build good habits & break bad ones.* New York, New York, Avery, an imprint of Penguin Random House.

I've seen people join the gym and do two hours a day, seven days a week. For most people, this is not sustainable and, three months later, they are no longer there. It is better to start small and consistent, build up slowly and be there 10 years later. This is much better than stopping after three months having peaked at your buff best self but never stepping foot in the gym or putting on your jogging shoes again.

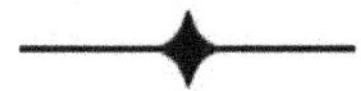

Starting Staggered

We often hear that it takes 21 days to break a bad habit or forge a new, good habit. We're now told it's more like three times that amount. Whether this is true or not, it makes sense that the longer you focus on a good habit you wish to form, it will certainly cement it more deeply in your mind, emotions and daily life. Based on this precept, below is one way you may wish to apply the current recommendations (mentioned in chapter 4) for exercise. Stagger start with one 'base movement', add resistance training and then, as you are getting fitter, ramp up the intensity. Of course, if you want to jump in, boots and all, go for it!

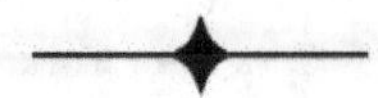

Overview

1. **Move:** Start building up your activity levels with basic walking. Create the habit. Even if it's five minutes at a time, just start. If you can't walk due to physical reasons (e.g., joint issues), then cycle or swim. Whatever you choose, make sure you are safe. Walking outdoors has loads of benefits, but if you cannot fit it in during daylight hours, a treadmill at the gym might be safer. Similarly, an upright bike at the gym may be safer than cycling on the road. Work out what will be best for you. Keep the intensity low to moderate at this stage.

   ➤ Add on some stretching. Try a couple of the stretches in Chapter 7.

2. **Resist:** Once you've got the habit of walking under your belt, add some resistance training. Start with one workout a week: e.g., a home-based workout in the next chapter, a program at a gym or a resistance-based class such as Pilates or a weights circuit.

   ➤ Add one to two balance exercises into your resistance training. See samples in Chapter 7.

3. ***Intensify:*** Now that you are feeling fitter and have strengthened your muscles, begin with adding some high-intensity cardio workouts. This might be as simple as adding some hills or jogging while you're walking (or quick bursts while you're cycling or swimming). Or you might like to add it as a separate workout with the purpose of raising your heart rate. There are many extra types of cardio equipment at the gym, e.g., stepper or cross trainer. Here, we are aiming for moderate to vigorous exercise.

Once you've started and are experiencing the benefits of exercise, aim to build up to the recommended levels of exercise as you become inspired and motivated. This will mean you are aiming for:

- ➤ Walking: Aiming to walk for 30 mins (or more) five times per week (include stretching)

- ➤ Resistance: Including at least two full body workouts per week (or split into muscle groups and spread over more days). (Add balance and stretching.)

- ➤ Intensity: Include some vigorous exercise in your cardio workouts. (More stretching.)

Walking Tips

Start with a good pair of walking shoes, as mentioned previously. This will protect your feet and cushion your joints. Stay safe if you are walking on the road beside cars. Try to walk on the side of the road where you are facing the oncoming traffic. This way, you can see it and get off the road if necessary. Listening to music and podcasts are a great way to make your walk more relaxing or inspiring, but make sure you can hear traffic if you are not on a footpath. Two cars can sound like one car, so always check before you step back onto the road.

CHAPTER 6

Epiphany Moments

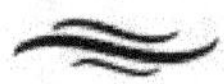

When I was a coffee-clutching couch dweller, I thought I knew stuff about exercise, but I've learnt way more by *doing* exercise. I'd like to share my epiphany moments with you with the hope that they will be helpful to set you on your exercise journey.

1. Start small – Start with what you can. As you get fitter, chances are you will inspire yourself to the next level!

2. Start simple – Don't make it complicated. Keep your exercise moments as barrier-free as possible.

3. Plan it– Hit the ground running by being organized so that you set yourself up for success (not failure).

4. Prioritise it – Schedule it into your week at a time slot where it won't be overtaken with something 'more important'. Going to the gym or a class after work? Pack your bag and leave it in the boot. Once you go home, chances are your motivation levels will drop.

5. Protect it – See it as an appointment where you can say, "Sorry, can't stay and chat, I have an appointment." No one knows it's an appointment with yourself at the gym. ☺

5. Enjoy it – Choose something that you enjoy enough to keep you coming back.

6. Vary it – If you start to get bored, set a goal, change the class you'rc going to or get a new program at the gym...

Well, that's plenty of information to get started.

CHAPTER 7

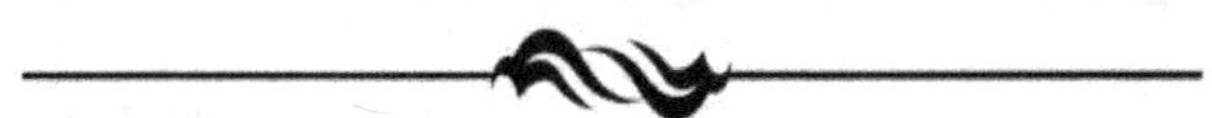

Workouts

I f you are not currently exercising, you should talk to your doctor before starting any exercise program. Particularly if you have the following conditions:

> Heart condition or stroke.

> Chest pains or discomfort during physical activity.

> Feel dizzy or faint or lose balance during activity.

> Have had an asthma attack requiring medical attention in the last 12 months.

> Have type 1 or 2 diabetes and have trouble controlling your blood pressure.

> ➢ Any other conditions that would make it difficult to exercise.

Fitness Levels

Following are some guidelines for performing these workouts at your fitness level. Make sure you leave a day in between so that you are not overworking the muscles. The process of 'repair' takes place in the 48 hours after the workout. This is where the muscle grows so that we can see the 'toned' result.

Beginners

- Attempt up to as many of the recommended repetitions ("reps") as you can for each exercise. Increase the number a little bit each time you do the circuit.

- Start with one exercise session per week so that you are not overly sore. Increase to two sessions when you are ready.

Intermediate

- Do two to three circuits of the program in each session.

- Aim to do an exercise session two or more times per week.

Advanced

- To advance this routine, you can move onto using dumbbells (DB) for the squats and lunges, but make sure you keep the correct form. Look for 'DB' in the exercises.

For Everyone

The four workouts are not necessarily graded from easy to increasing difficulty. They are simply put together as four different options for a balanced, full-body workout. You might want to stay with one workout for four weeks, or you might want to vary between each of them. You will be able to track your progress more if you stick with one workout for a month. But it's also good to keep your muscles guessing by changing to different exercises, so move onto a new circuit after 4 to 6 weeks.

If you're using new muscle groups, you may experience DOMS (delayed onset muscle soreness). To minimize this, start small, e.g., just one round of the circuit instead of three. Keep stretching after your workouts.

Breathing: In general, exhale on the hardest part of the movement (the 'push', 'pull', 'lift' phases) and inhale on the return phase.

1. Home-Based No Equipment Circuit 1

Exercise	Body part	Repetitions and Form	Diagram
Push-up	Chest and biceps	1-10 From a plank position (knees or toes), take your hands wider than your shoulders. Bend at the elbows to lower to the ground, and then push up. To protect your lower back, engage abs, lifting your belly button away from the floor.	or from the knees
Squats	Quadriceps	1-10 Start with your feet hip distance apart. Bend at the knees with the weight in your heels more than your toes. Your knees should track in line with your toes.	
Plank from hands	Abs	10-30 seconds When you are planking, aim to be in a long, straight line (i.e., not piking or sagging) to	(also on knees)

Exercise	Body part	Repetitions and Form	Diagram
		protect your lower back. Engage your abs, thinking about drawing your belly button away from the floor.	
Static lunges	Hamstrings	1-10 (each leg) Step one foot out in front, but still hip distance apart. Bend both legs in a downward motion. Keep the front knee above your toes (rather than going forward past them). Repeat all reps on one leg, then switch to the other leg.	(Advanced: Add DB)
Superman hold	Glutes and back	10-30 seconds Start lying on your stomach, arms straight and stretched overhead. Squeeze glutes and shoulder blades as you lift both arms and legs off the floor. Continue to hold, remembering to breathe.	

Exercise	Body part	Repetitions and Form	Diagram
Balance	Heel-to-toe walk. In a clear area, place the heel of one foot directly in front of the other and repeat. Look up to make it more challenging.		

---

2. Home-Based No Equipment Circuit 2

Exercise	Body part	Repetitions and Form	Diagram
Tricep dips	Triceps	1-10 Place a chair against a wall. Sit on it and place your hands next to you. Push up off the chair so your butt is in front of the chair. Bend your elbows to lower your body down and then push up into a straight arm. Continue. Legs bent is easier; legs straight is harder.	
Wide-leg squats	Quadriceps	1-10 Place your legs out wide, feet turned out. Squat down. Your knees should travel out in line you're your toes. Have more of your weight on your heels than your toes.	

Exercise	Body part	Repetitions and Form	Diagram
Side plank from hand or forearm	Oblique abs	10–30 seconds (each side) From the knees or toes, hold up in a side plank. Think about drawing the side of your waist away from the floor. Keep your shoulders and hips facing forward, rather than rotating to the ground. This can also be done from your forearm instead of hand.	
Hip lifts (with or without band)	Glutes and hamstrings	1–10 Lying on your back, knees bent. Push your hips up, digging your heels into the mat to engage your glutes more. Keep your abs switched on to protect your lower back. Lower hips down and repeat.	

Exercise	Body part	Repetitions and Form	Diagram
T-lifts	Back	1-10 Lying on your stomach on the ground, stretch both arms out at right angles to the body and lift up and down.	
Balance		One leg stand (30 seconds on each leg).	

3. Home-Based Workout with Resistance Band Circuit 1

Exercise	Body part	Repetitions and Form	Diagram
Tricep push-ups	Triceps	1-10 Place hands shoulder-distance apart (i.e., not as wide as a regular push-up). Keep elbows pointing back rather than out. It is harder than a regular push-up, so you may need to go on your knees.	
Hinge	Quadriceps	1-10 Begin kneeling on a mat. Arms straight out in front. Lean back slightly, then move forward. Try not to bend at the hips or sway your back. Legs and torso should stay in one straight line. You do not need to lean back very far to feel this in the front of your thighs.	

Exercise	Body part	Repetitions and Form	Diagram
Ab crunch	Abs	1-10 Lying on your back with your knees bent, feel on the floor. Reach your hands up or cross them over your chest. Tuck your chin and curl up so that the bottom of your ribs gets closer to your hips. Control on the way back. Repeat.	
Step out squat	Quads/hams /glutes	1-10 Perform a normal squat (feet hip distance apart). Step to one side (the other leg stays where it is). Perform a wide-leg squat. Repeat a normal squat; step to the other side and perform a wide-leg squat. One rep is both sides.	
Bicep Curl with band	Biceps	1-10 Sitting on the floor, legs extended out in front with a slight bend. Place the band in your arches. Lock	

Exercise	Body part	Repetitions and Form	Diagram
		your elbows near your ribs and draw your thumbs toward your shoulders.	
Row with band	Back	1-10 Sitting on the floor, legs extended straight. Draw the band back so that your elbows extend back past your ribs. Squeeze your shoulder blades together. Release the band with control and repeat.	
Moving Balance		Stand on one leg. With the other foot, tap your ankle, mid-calf and knee; then reverse. Do this for 30 seconds on each leg.	

4. Home Based Workout with Resistance Band Circuit 2

Exercise	Body part	Repetitions and Form	Diagram
Rear Delt Fly's with band	Back/chest	1-10 Stand with abs engaged and a slight bend in the knees. Holding band at armpit level, pull the band apart so that it stretches. Squeeze shoulder blades together. Release band with control, repeat. To make it harder, keep tension on the band at all times so that it does not go slack.	
Alternating lunges	Hams/glutes	1-10 (each leg) Lunge forward with one leg, bending both legs and keeping the front knee above the toes. Return up, swap legs and lunge down again. Keep alternating your legs (this is	(Advanced: Add DB)

Exercise	Body part	Repetitions and Form	Diagram
		different from the static lunges).	
Bicycle abs	Abs	1-10 (each leg) Start on your back on a mat, knees bent. Place hands behind your head and lift your upper body up off the ground. Rotate torso to one side and draw the opposite knee to elbow. Repeat the other way (this is one rep).	
Calf raises	Calves	1-20 Starting with flat feet, then lift heels up and down.	
Lateral raises with band	Shoulders	1-10 Place the centre of the band under your feet. Engage your abs and have a slight bend in your knees. With almost straight arms, pull the band up beside your body (not in	

Exercise	Body part	Repetitions and Form	Diagram
		front). Release down and repeat.	
Balance		Stand on one leg (eyes closed). Stay near a wall or sturdy object that you can grab onto if needed. Hands up as shown will be more difficult. You can choose to have your hands down to begin with if you prefer.	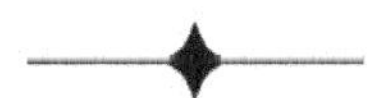

Stretching

You can do these at the end of your Movement, Resistance or Intensify sessions. Hold for 30 seconds, or as long as comfortable. Aim for an intensity level of about 6-7 out of 10. Stop/ease back if you feel shaky or faint when stretching.

Stretch Name	Body Part being Stretched	Diagram
Kneeling hip flexor stretch	Hip flexor (front of hip) This can also be done alongside a chair if you'd prefer not to kneel	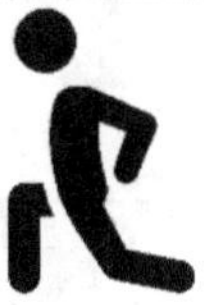 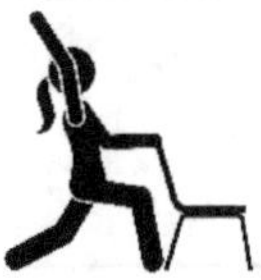
Hamstring stretch	Hamstring (back of thigh)	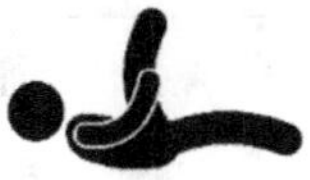
Chest stretch	Chest, front shoulder and bicep	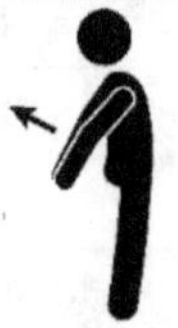
Tricep stretch	Triceps–back of arm	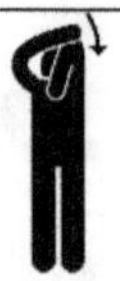
Standing quad stretch	Front of thigh	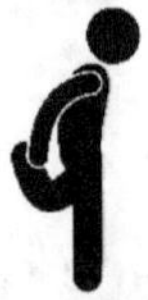
Shoulder stretch	Mid and rear shoulder	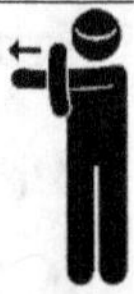
Candlestick stretch	Side of torso	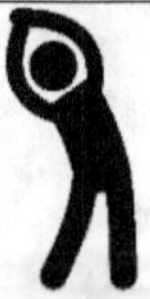

Stretch Name	Body Part being Stretched	Diagram
Prayer stretch	Back and recovery position	
Runner's stretch	Back of thigh, calf, front of hip	

CHAPTER 8

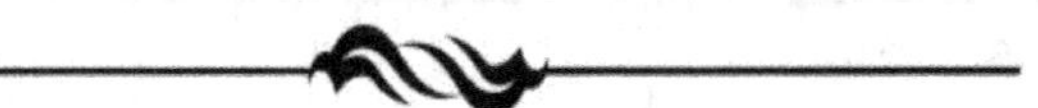

Training Schedules

Following is a set of schedules where you can track your progress over nine weeks. There are some extra schedules included for those who may wish to jump straight into resistance and vigorous exercise.

1. Base Movement. We are aiming for 30 minutes of exercise but start where you need to, even if it's five minutes. Track your minutes walked so you can slowly add a bit more and look back and seeing your progress. You do not have to walk every day but try to walk most days or at least every second day. However, try to

factor in one day off so that your body can recover and to give you a mental break.

2. Resist: If you are new to exercise, even though you have already completed the three weeks of 'Moving', you may want to start with one session and build up to two. Start where you need to, e.g., five minutes or 'one rep'– do whatever you need to so that you keep coming back for more.

3. Intensify: As your fitness has now increased through moving and resistance training, begin to add vigorous exercise. Sprints, HIIT classes, jogging, walking up hills, etc. Attending a 'cardio' style class can also help to include more vigorous exercise in your week. This includes spin (cycle) classes, HIIT-based classes and boot camps.

1. Move (walk, cycle or swim)

> ➤ Aim to move (e.g., walk, cycle or swim) for 30 mins (or more), five times per week (and stretch at the end). It's ok to start with five minutes of moving and work up to more.

WEEK 1	Date	Mins Walked	Mins Stretched
Monday			
Tuesday			
Wednesday			
Thursday			
Friday			
Saturday			
Sunday			
TOTALS:			

How did it feel? What did you enjoy? What did you dislike?

Continue moving, adding a bit more this week if you are not yet doing 30 minutes.

WEEK 2	Date	Mins Walked	Mins Stretched
Monday			
Tuesday			
Wednesday			
Thursday			
Friday			
Saturday			
Sunday			
TOTALS:			

How did it feel? What did you enjoy? What did you dislike?

It's week three, keep moving. Maybe you're starting to lose motivation? Go back and read your 'why' and say your positive affirmations out loud. Think about what you may need to rearrange in your schedule to prioritise your health.

WEEK 3	Date	Mins Walked	Mins Stretched
Monday			
Tuesday			
Wednesday			
Thursday			
Friday			
Saturday			
Sunday			
TOTALS:			

How did it feel? What did you enjoy? What did you dislike?

2. Resist: Start to include at least one to two full-body workouts per week. This can be the circuits in this book, your own program at home or in the gym, or a resistance-based fitness class (as opposed to cardio). If you are doing your own programs, don't forget to add one or two balance exercises.

WEEK 4	Date	Mins Walked	Mins Stretched	Mins Resistance	Mins Balance
Monday					
Tuesday					
Wednesday					
Thursday					
Friday					
Saturday					
Sunday					
TOTALS:					

How did it feel? What did you enjoy? What did you dislike?

It's week 5. You may have experienced some muscle soreness after adding in resistance training last week. The first week is usually the sorest. Start to add another round of the circuit.

WEEK 5	Date	Mins Walked	Mins Stretched	Mins Resistance	Mins Balance
Monday					
Tuesday					
Wednesday					
Thursday					
Friday					
Saturday					
Sunday					
TOTALS:					

How did it feel? What did you enjoy? What did you dislike?

By now, you will be powering into your resistance training. Or if you've missed a session or two, it's a new week—resolve to start again. Schedule your best times to add resistance training into your week and protect it! If you're following the workouts in this book, try the full three circuits.

WEEK 6	Date	Mins Walked	Mins Stretched	Mins Resistance	Mins Balance
Monday					
Tuesday					
Wednesday					
Thursday					
Friday					
Saturday					
Sunday					
TOTALS:					

How did it feel? What did you enjoy? What did you dislike?

3. *Intensify*: It's time to include some vigorous exercise in your cardio workouts or schedule them at a separate time. You can do this by adding in some hills to your walking or cycling, adding in some 20-30 seconds sprints, or doing it at a separate place from your base movement. This may be the most challenging part of your exercising, but it's got the 'feel good' benefits. Take note of how you feel after your session.

WEEK 7	Date	Mins Moved	Mins Stretched	Mins Resistance	Mins Balance	Mins Intensity
Monday						
Tuesday						
Wednesday						
Thursday						
Friday						
Saturday						
Sunday						
TOTALS						

How did it feel? What did you enjoy? What did you dislike?

Wow, week 8. Look how far you've come! Keep it up. You may think about what type of vigorous exercise is working best for you—including it in your walking or a separate session. Journal your way to the best plan for you.

WEEK 8	Date	Mins Moved	Mins Stretched	Mins Resistance	Mins Balance	Mins Intensity
Monday						
Tuesday						
Wednesday						
Thursday						
Friday						
Saturday						
Sunday						
TOTALS						

How did it feel? What did you enjoy? What did you dislike?

By now, you will be feeling fit and reaping the benefits. You're creating new habits to set yourself up for better health, energy, confidence and more. Keep tweaking your schedule so that you build exercise into your life in a way that works for you.

WEEK 9	Date	Mins Moved	Mins Stretched	Mins Resistance	Mins Balance	Mins Intensity
Monday						
Tuesday						
Wednesday						
Thursday						
Friday						
Saturday						
Sunday						
TOTALS						

How did it feel? What did you enjoy? What did you dislike?

Congratulations! Be proud of yourself. You have completed nine weeks of activity. It's not easy to change habits, but now that you have broken through the initial barriers, it will be easier to sustain.

Here are another three weeks so you can keep tracking your progress:

WEEK 10	Date	Mins Moved	Mins Stretched	Mins Resistance	Mins Balance	Mins Intensity
Monday						
Tuesday						
Wednesday						
Thursday						
Friday						
Saturday						
Sunday						
TOTALS						

WEEK 11	Date	Mins Moved	Mins Stretched	Mins Resistance	Mins Balance	Mins Intensity
Monday						
Tuesday						
Wednesday						
Thursday						
Friday						
Saturday						
Sunday						
TOTALS						

WEEK 12	Date	Mins Moved	Mins Stretched	Mins Resistance	Mins Balance	Mins Intensity
Monday						
Tuesday						
Wednesday						
Thursday						
Friday						
Saturday						
Sunday						
TOTALS						

CHAPTER 9

Re-Write Your Story

Now that you have spent many weeks carving our good, life-giving habits, what is your story? Has it changed from the story you wrote in Chapter 1? Hopefully, you now have a new identity around exercise. If you have worked through the guidelines in the workbook, you can now confidently say, "I am someone who lives an active lifestyle." This is your new identity. Keep proving to yourself that that is who you are.

Re-Activate Your Who

Who are you when it comes to exercise? If it was a relationship, how would you describe it? Circle one below that fits you best right now:

Unacquainted	Distant acquaintance	Casual friendship
Friend	Close friend	Long-term relationship
	It's complicated!	

What is your exercise experience now? Below (or in a notebook), take a few minutes to think about how your relationship with exercise has changed since you started getting off the couch. Celebrate your successes; write about how getting active has benefited your life; where has it been challenged? What are your goals going forward?

If you'd like to continue tracking your workouts, you can purchase the following journal:

Move, Resist, Intensify

Fitness Tracker

APPENDIX

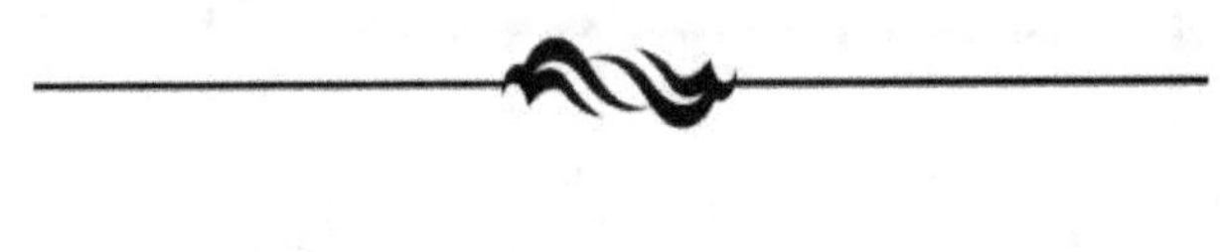

Heart Rate Zones

Intensity levels are an individual thing. A super fit person may not get into the vigorous zone until they walk up a steep hill or go on a fast run. Someone unused to exercise may get their heart rate quite high just by walking on flat ground. Comparisons with someone else will be inaccurate. Using the intensity levels mentioned in Chapter 4 are an easy way to work out what level you're walking at. However, there are calculations as well. Fitbits and smartwatches are probably the easiest methods. Here are the calculations:

- ➢ Moderate Intensity: 60% of your maximum heart rate
- ➢ Vigorous Intensity: 70% or more of your maximum heart rate

You can calculate your maximum heart rate as follows:

Maximum Heart Rate ("MHR"):

- ➢ 220 – AGE = _ _ _ _ _ _
- ➢ 70% MHR = _ _ _ _ _ _
- ➢ 60% = _ _ _ _ _ _

Resting Heart Rate ("RHR")

As you get fitter, your 'resting heart rate' will get lower. In general, a lower heart rate (normal is between 40 and 100) is better as it means your heart is working more efficiently.

The best time to measure your resting heart rate is first thing in the morning before you get out of bed. If you do not have a smartwatch that tracks this, place your middle and index finger on the inside of your wrist (on the thumb side), or under your jaw. Find your pulse and time it for 15 seconds and multiply it by four to get the total per minute (or just count it for a minute).

You might find it interesting to track this as you progress in your exercise. It will be encouraging to see it go down. The above heart rate calculation is based on the general population. If you want to find a more specific way of calculating your 60% and 70% zones, you can Google the Karvonen method, which uses your resting heart rate as the basis of the calculation rather than the general population.

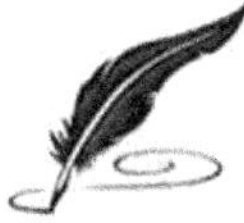

About the Author

Robyn lives in a small rural town in northern NSW, Australia. She currently works at the local community gym, instructing Pilates and other classes. Her qualifications include fitness, Pilates, group exercise, weight management, nutrition, wellness and counselling. Robyn is passionate about the role of exercise and nutrition in longevity—living well for longer.

References

https://www.sciencedirect.com/science/article/pii/S037851221
7308563

https://www.sciencedirect.com/science/article/pii/S002561961
1652191

https://www.health.gov.au/health-topics/physical-activity-and-exercise/physical-activity-and-exercise-guidelines-for-all-australians/for-adults-18-to-64-years:

https://pubmed.ncbi.nlm.nih.gov/16377300/ Swain DP, Franklin BA. Comparison of cardioprotective benefits of vigorous versus moderate intensity aerobic exercise. Am J Cardiol. 2006 Jan 1;97(1):141-7. doi: 10.1016/j.amjcard .2005.07.130. Epub 2005 Nov 16. PMID: 16377300.

Clear, J. (2018). *Atomic habits: tiny changes, remarkable results : an easy & proven way to build good habits & break bad ones.* New York, New York, Avery, an imprint of Penguin Random House.